Author

Keith D. DeDonder

DVM, MSc, PhD

Graduated from Kansas State University College of Veterinary Medicine, the focus of his PhD research was on antimicrobial resistance in bovine respiratory disease (BRD) and the effects of clinical BRD on the pharmacokinetics and pharmacodynamics of an antibiotic and its correlation to treatment outcome. He is now director of clinical services at the Veterinary and Biomedical Research Center in the United States providing quality research to the veterinary and biomedical community.

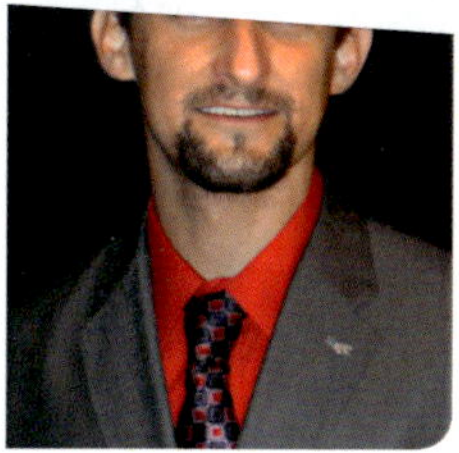

TABLE OF CONTENTS

Introduction and global importance

BRDC is a major worldwide disease affecting the cattle industry. It continues to be an economic drain globally due to lost animal production, increased labour expense, the cost of drugs used in treatment, and mortality. One North American author estimated the economic impact of BRDC globally to be in excess of $1 billion US dollars annually in the feedlot industry alone. [1] BRDC is the number one cause of morbidity and mortality in young, intensely raised cattle. [2]

Many factors contribute and are responsible for the continued struggle with BRDC. It is a complex, multi-factorial disease with several bacterial and viral agents often implicated which are precipitated by stressful events.

Table 1. Non-exhaustive list of stressors, viral pathogens and bacterial pathogens most often indicated as the agents or events that often lead up to BRDC. The most commonly cited scenario is a stressful event causing immunosuppression leading to viral invasion and secondary bacterial colonization.

Stressors	Viral pathogens	Bacterial pathogens
Transport. Weaning. Processing. Weather extremes. Commingling.	Bovine viral diarrhoea virus. Bovine respiratory syncytial virus. Bovine herpes virus. Parainfluenza virus-3.	*Mannheimia haemolytica.* *Pasteurella multocida.* *Histophilus somni.* *Mycoplasma bovis.*

It is difficult to accurately diagnose BRDC due to the occurrence of non-specific clinical signs, lack of a gold-standard diagnostic test, and the fact that cattle are a prey species and therefore hide signs of disease from the observer. Cattle are anatomically and physiologically predisposed to the development of pulmonary disease. In comparison to other farm animal species, cattle have a decreased gaseous exchange capacity, lower alveolar oxygen levels during high metabolic activity, decreased pulmonary clearance, and a greater degree of compartmentalization all of which leads to a reduced phagocytic activity and a more favourable environment for infectious agents. [3]

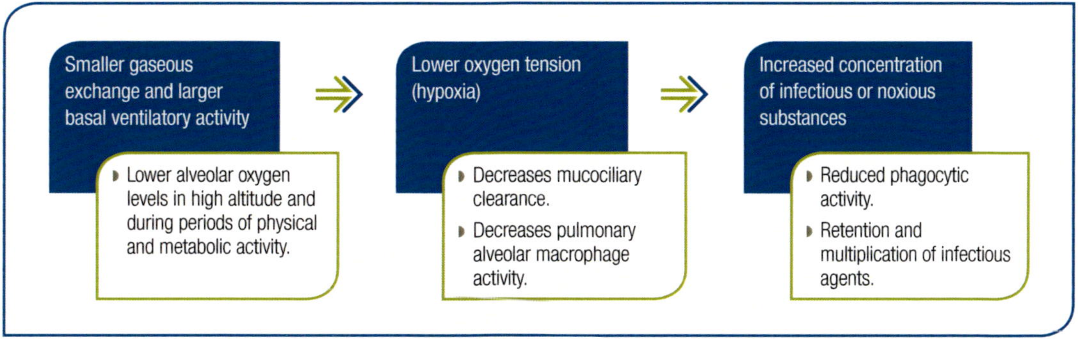

Figure 1. Anatomical and physiological features owing to a relative predisposition of the bovine lung to developing BRDC. The higher degree of the compartmentalization, leading to microenvironments of hypoxic and occluded airways, lead to a predisposition for pulmonary lesions typical of BRDC.[3]

Types of disease

Broadly defined, respiratory disease would include any process causing pathology to the respiratory system. In cattle there are many diseases that can induce respiratory system pathology including acute interstitial pneumonia (also termed atypical interstitial pneumonia), lungworms, aspiration pneumonia, calf diphtheria, etc. Additionally, BRDC has many synonyms that further confuse the situation including shipping fever, pasteurellosis, pneumonia, bronchopneumonia, and fibrous pleuropneumonia, among others. However, the context referred to as BRDC is a pneumonia, acute or chronic, caused by an infectious agent with associated inflammation (often suppurative and fibrous).

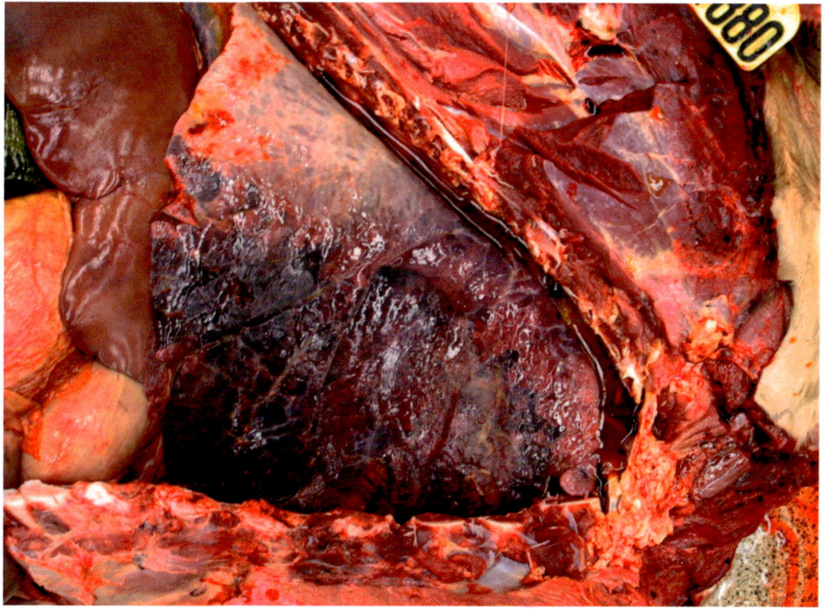

Figure 2. Severe, advanced lung lesions in a calf that succumbed to BRDC. The ventral lung fields are severely consolidated, with only a small (caudal and dorsal) portion of lung remaining. Also noticeable are areas of fibrin (hazy white on surface) accumulation.

As previously detailed, the contemporary cascade leading to BRDC is a mixture of stressors leading to immunosuppression, followed by a viral invasion of the upper and lower respiratory tract (URT/LRT) leading to further immunosuppression and mucosal injury, with subsequent bacterial infection.[4-6] The most common viruses and bacteria implicated in this cascade are the focus of this chapter.

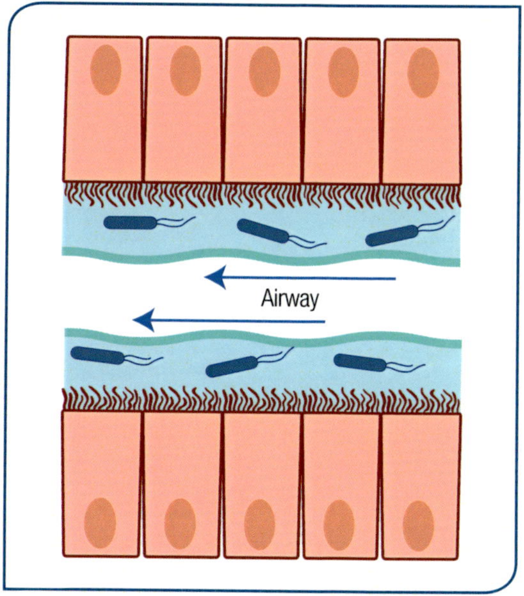

Figure 3. The mucociliary tree lines the airways and normally clears particles and pathogens from the airways using a "lift" effect by pushing them out of the airways and out of the body via mucous.

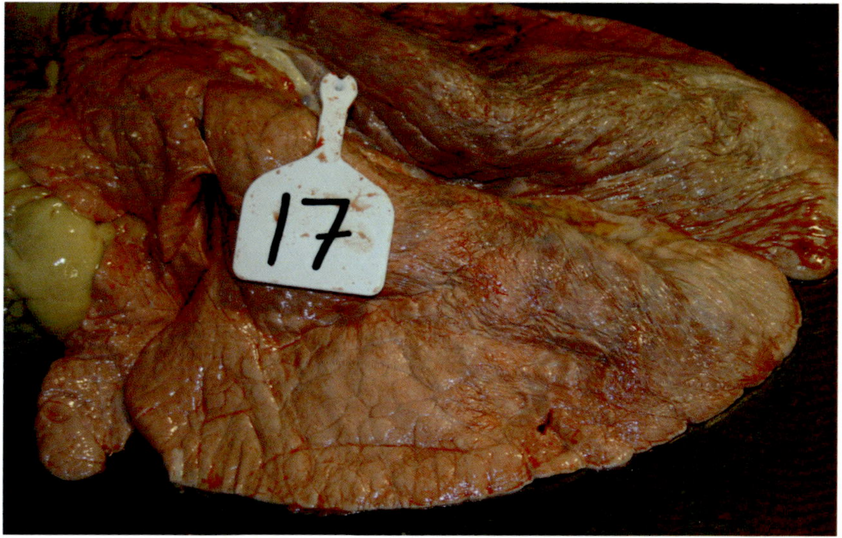

Figure 4. Normal lungs, no pathology present. Notice the healthy pink colour and how the lung is collapsed and spongy in appearance and feel.

Common viral agents

General viral pathogenesis includes damage to the mucosal lining, induced immunosuppression, decreased mucociliary clearance, depressed phagocytic activity, and phagocytic cell death.[5,7] The decreased immune function and build-up of fluid and cellular debris in the airways produce an excellent medium for bacterial cell proliferation.

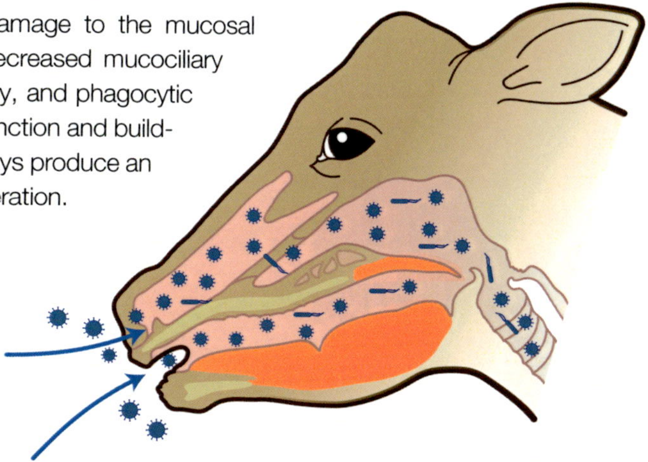

Figure 5. Viruses enter via the nose/mouth and damage the mucosa, decreasing mucociliary clearance and causing generalized immunosuppression. Bacteria are inhaled from the URT into the LRT and proliferate.

Bovine diarrhoea virus (BVDV)

BVDV has been extensively studied and many experiments have shown that BVDV works in synergy with other pathogens and exacerbates lesions of BRDC.[8, 9] BVDV is one of the most immunosuppressive viruses, but alone is generally not a primary cause of BRDC and does not cause specific lesions.[10] However, calves infected *in utero* with non-cytopathic strains between 40-125 days of gestation become carriers of the virus (persistent infection) and shed it in large numbers throughout their lives. These persistently infected cattle are much more likely to die from BVDV than those with acute infection. However, they can maintain a healthy status which makes them difficult to identify without diagnostic testing.

Bovine respiratory syncytial virus (BRSV)

Infections from BRSV occur primarily in young naïve beef and dairy calves, and can result in severe respiratory disease. Pyrexia, anorexia, increased respiratory rate, cough, nasal and lacrimal discharge, and dyspnoea (e.g. open-mouthed breathing) are all clinical signs associated with BRSV. BRSV has a greater potential for lethal respiratory disease as a lone pathogen than the other viruses of BRDC. Necropsy lesions include moderate cranioventral, red consolidation with a lobular pattern and emphysematous caudodorsal lung fields. [10]

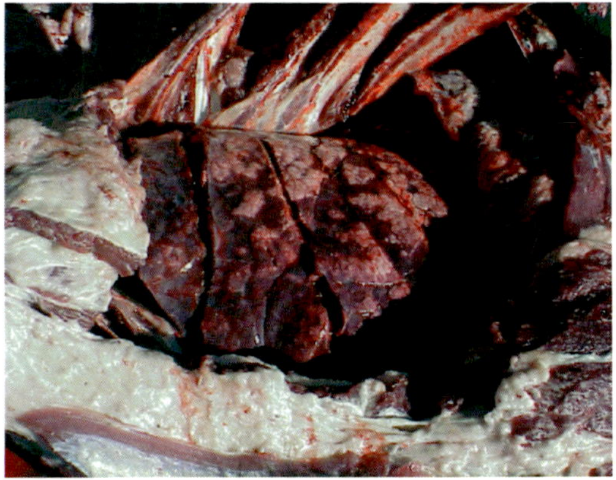

Figure 6. Lesions typical of BRSV: cranioventral, red consolidation with a lobular pattern; severe cases will display emphysema of the caudodorsal lung.

Bovine herpes virus (BHV)

BHV type 1 is the causative agent of infectious bovine rhinotracheitis which typically causes pyrexia, anorexia, coughing, salivation, nasal discharge, conjunctivitis, inflamed nares, and dyspnoea if the larynx becomes occluded with purulent material.[10] The distinguishing characteristic of all herpes viruses; it establishes a latent infection in the trigeminal ganglion and can recrudesce in times of stress. However, disease is typically mild and self-limiting if not accompanied by other viral or bacterial pathogens.

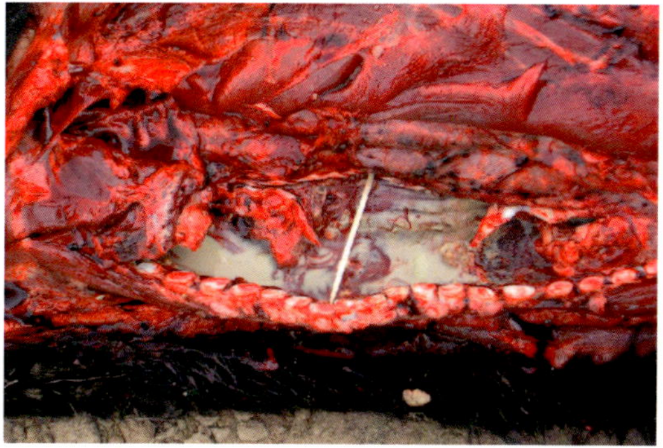

Figure 7. Characteristic lesion of BHV-1: severe mucopurulent and fibrinous tracheitis.

Parainfluenza virus-3 (PI3)

On rare occasions, PI3 can cause severe respiratory disease, but most infections result in a very mild disease of little concern. In naïve cattle or co-infection, the virus can cause a rhinitis with mucopurulent exudate in the nares and experimentally induced infection can cause atelectasis and consolidation.[10]

Bovine respiratory coronavirus (BRCV)

Reports of outbreaks caused by BRCV infections have been reported, but a direct link between viral infection and causation of disease has not been established.[11]

Common bacterial agents

Bacteria are considered to be secondary invaders subsequent to viral invasion, but can also be primary pathologic agents.[10] The bacteria implicated in BRDC are normal inhabitants of the URT and gain access to the LRT via inhalation of droplets or biofilms.[10, 12, 13] The majority of the damage done to the lungs is from the bacterial component of the infection and the ensuing inflammation.

Mannheimia haemolytica (MH)

- MH is considered by many to be the primary bacterial pathogen associated with BRDC. It is a gram-negative, facultative anaerobic bacterium.[7] MH is a commensal bacterium, but has been shown to directly cause lesions and death by inoculation into the lungs and thoracic cavity.[7]
- In the past, classification schemes, such as serotyping, have been used to differentiate strains of MH. However, DNA sequencing techniques might soon replace these methods and are allowing researchers to group MH in more specific subtypes which may allow great advancement in understanding the spread of bacteria within and between cattle populations.[14]

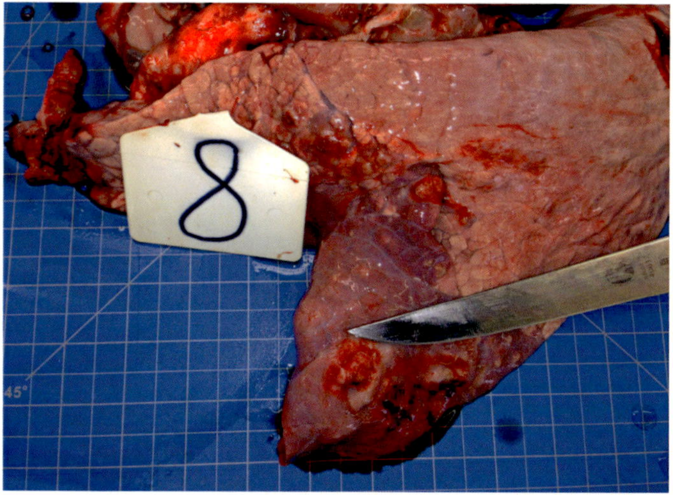

Figure 8. Cranioventral pneumonia with consolidation; dark cherry red lesions are considered by some to be a trademark of MH. This calf was euthanized 7 days after experimental infection with pure MH culture.

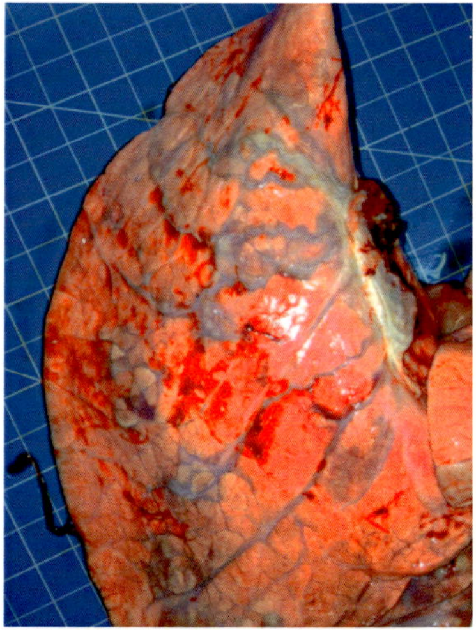

Figure 9. Another MH experimental infection showing interlobular pattern due to oedema that is often present on necropsy.

Pasteurella multocida (PM)

PM is a gram-negative commensal bacterium of the bovine URT and is commonly cultured from the nares and nasopharyngeal swabs in healthy cattle.[7] It is traditionally considered to be of less importance in BRDC as compared to MH. However, the isolation of PM from cases of BRDC are becoming more common place[7, 15] and some publications even cite PM as the most important BRDC pathogen.[16]

Histophilus somni (HS)

HS is a gram-negative commensal bacterium of the bovine URT, but may preferentially colonize the LRT.[7] HS is associated with BRDC, but can also cause a variety of other pathological processes such as septicaemia, synovitis, thrombotic meningoencephalomyelitis (TEME), fibrinous pericarditis, and sudden death associated with left ventricular papillary muscle necrosis.[5, 15] The reported prevalence of HS in samples of BRDC specimens varies, but its detection in field cases is typically lower than that of MH and PM, partially due to it being a more fastidious organism to culture.

Mycoplasma bovis (MB)

- MB is a unique bacterium as compared to MH, PM and HS. MB does not have a cell wall but, instead, it has a membrane which has implications in antimicrobial therapy selection. The importance of MB in BRDC is heavily debated. The causal relationship is not as clear for MB as for the other three bacteria on whether or not MB is a primary pathogen or just an opportunistic inhabitant of chronic BRD.[7]

- However, MB does play a role in BRDC +/- associated otitis media, and can also cause arthritis and tenosynovitis, among other diseases, and its prevalence in BRDC samples varies by geographical region.[17, 18] Depending on the detection techniques, MB is often not found on nasal swabs of healthy animals, but is more often found in LRT samples. Upon initial infection, MB is well known to persist due to the difficulty in antimicrobial cure and immune evasion and is therefore often present in samples of chronic BRD cases.

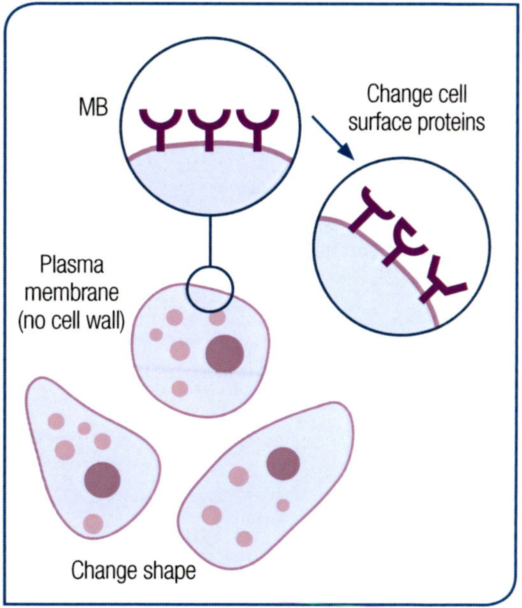

Figure 10. MB lacks a true cell wall and is thus able to change shape, to be inherently resistant to some antibiotics, to change cell surface proteins, and its size (0.2-0.8 μm) allows it to easily distribute around the body.

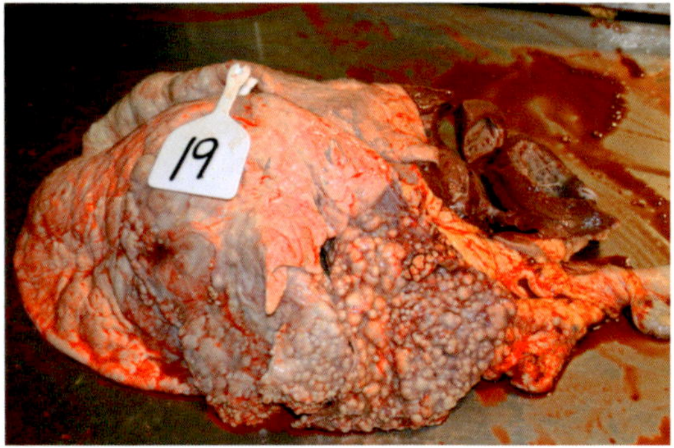

Figure 11. Severe cranioventral consolidation and abscessation typical of MB infection. Infections are very chronic in nature.

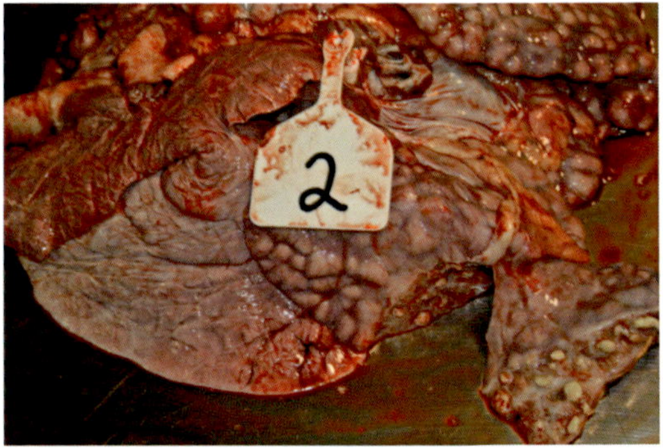

Figure 12. In cross section, the MB abscesses are visualized as caseous to inspissated.

Other bacteria

There are reports of other bacteria isolated from lungs of cattle with BRDC. Some of the more commonly reported bacteria include *Trueperella* (*Arcanobacterium*) *pyogenes*, *Bibersteinia trehalosi* and *Mannheimia varigena*. Some argue these organisms may be opportunistic pathogens or the result of chronic cases with prolonged antimicrobial therapy.

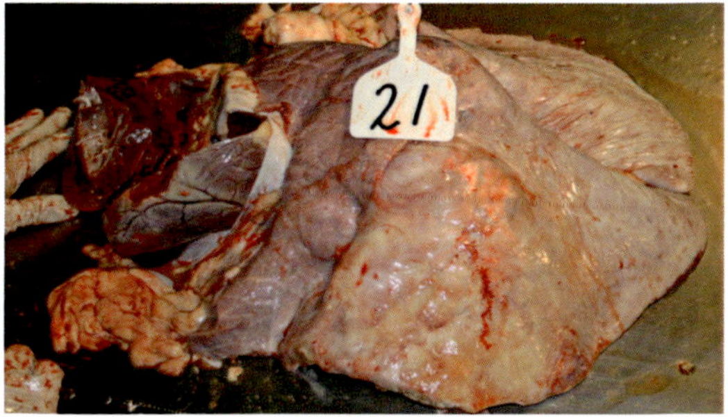

Figure 13. The glazy yellow film over the parietal surface is fibrin, often noted on necropsy. Notice the "full" appearance of the area covered in fibrin, heavy with consolidation.

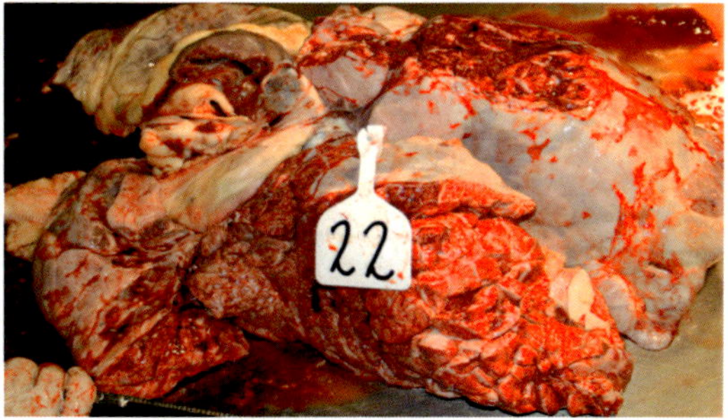

Figure 14. A "tear out" lesion at necropsy; the result of fibrous adhesions is so diffuse that the lung tears on removal from the thoracic cavity.

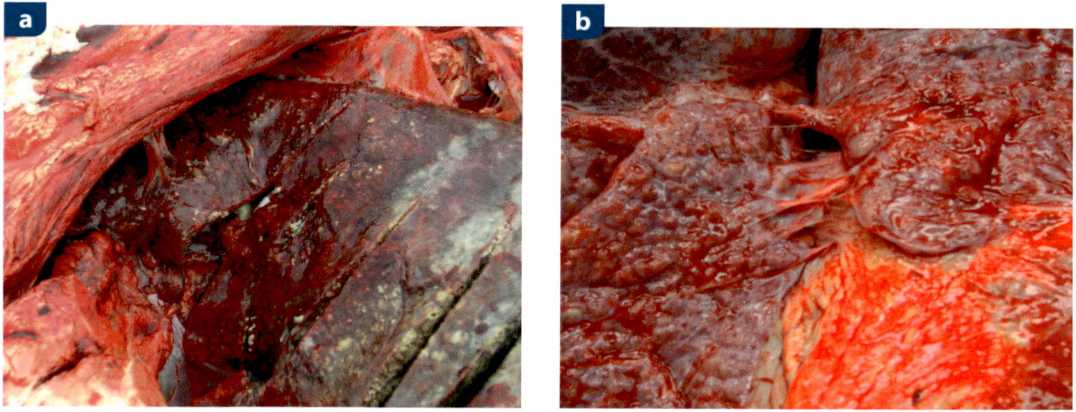

Figure 15. Very chronic case of BRDC displaying a fibrous tag between (a) the lung and the thoracic wall, and (b) two lung lobes.

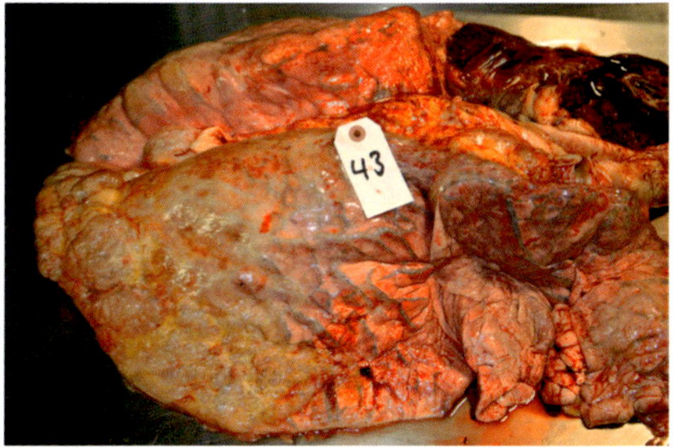

Figure 16. Severe, diffuse interlobular emphysema and oedema, large areas of fibrin accumulation. Interstitial emphysema is the result of laboured breathing, forcing air in the interstitial areas.

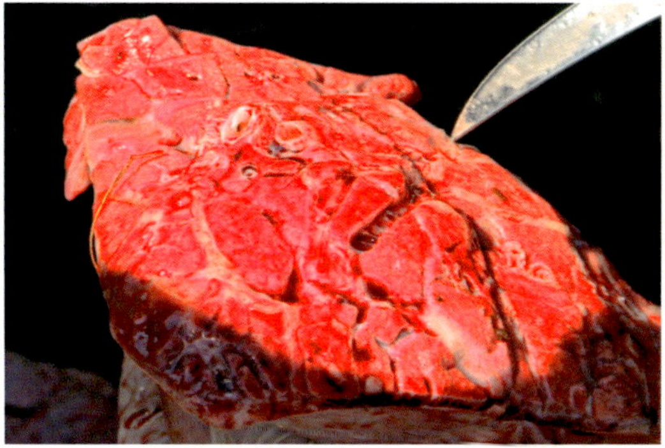

Figure 17. Cross section of lung with lobular pattern, consolidation, and interlobular emphysema and oedema. Image courtesy of Dr. DJ Rezac and Beef Cattle Institute.

Disease spread

- The spread of viral pathogens of BRDC is relatively well described. The primary means of viral spread is by nasal inhalation of aerosols or by direct contact with nasal secretions laden with virus.[19] Therefore, the introduction of an infected animal into a herd, or the confinement of cattle in pens could result in the spreading of viruses. In the case of BHV, stress can cause recrudescence, shedding of the virus from nasal secretions and subsequent spread of the infection between pen mates. Similarly, animals persistently infected with BVDV shed virus throughout their life and can serve as a factory for virus production.
- The epidemiology of bacterial spread in cattle populations is not as clear. There are conflicting reports that either support[20,21] or rebut[22,23] the hypothesis of direct animal-to-animal spread of the bacterial pathogens common to BRDC.

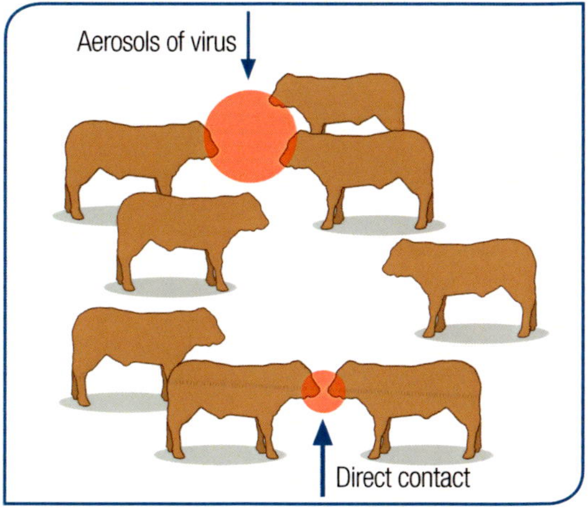

Figure 18. Viral pathogens of BRDC are spread by direct contact and aerosols of virus between pen mates.

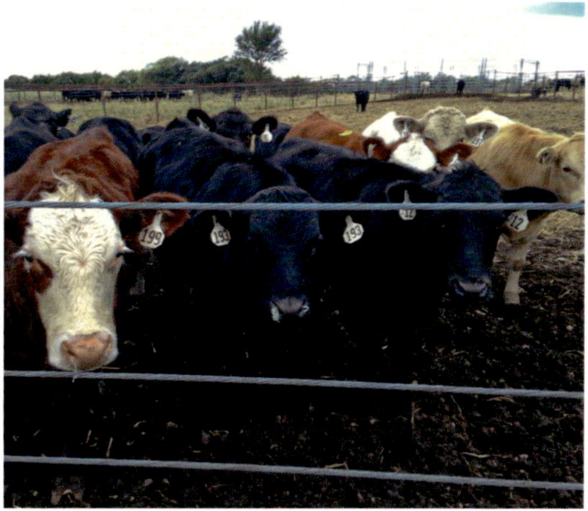

Figure 19. Viruses (and possibly bacteria) are shed in nasal secretions and can be spread directly or indirectly on shared fencing, bunk space, and water. This calf is draining purulent discharge onto the fence line.

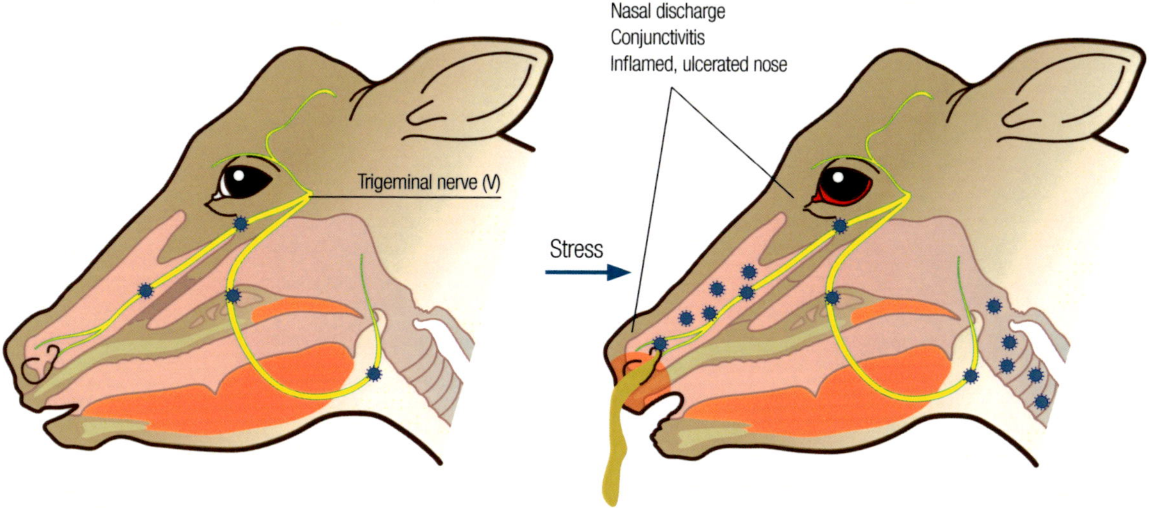

Figure 20. BHV infection results in a latent infection in the trigeminal ganglion that can recrudesce in times of stress and cause shedding of virus and infection of pen mates.

Management practices

- There are many stressors potentially involved in the pathogenesis of BRDC, often termed predisposing factors. However, there is little evidence of an actual association between these factors and the outcome (BRDC). In an exhaustive review of the literature, the only conclusive predisposing factors reported were that calves are at most risk of developing BRDC after transport/arrival to a fattening facility, with higher risks given to those cattle that went through an auction market and being commingled from multiple sources/herds. [24]

- In an epidemiological retrospective study in France, a cumulative incidence of BRDC at the farm level was reported to be around 10 % with the production type (increased in dairy) and herd size being noted as risk factors; BRDC was more common in the colder months, and cases of BRDC tended to cluster in space and time which was suggestive of a common infectious agent.[25]
- In a similar report of surveying producers, North American researchers found BRDC more common in cold months, an association with herd size and with the introduction of new calves into the herd.[26]

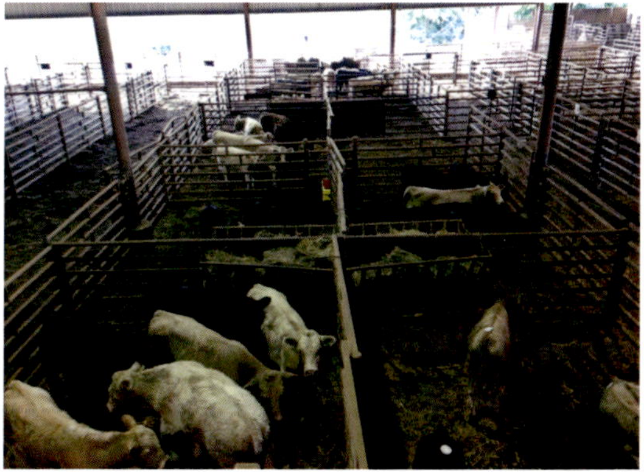

Figure 21. Cattle moving through auction markets are often commingled from many sources, share pen space and have ample opportunity for spread of disease between infected and naïve cattle. Image courtesy of Dr. Sarah Capik.

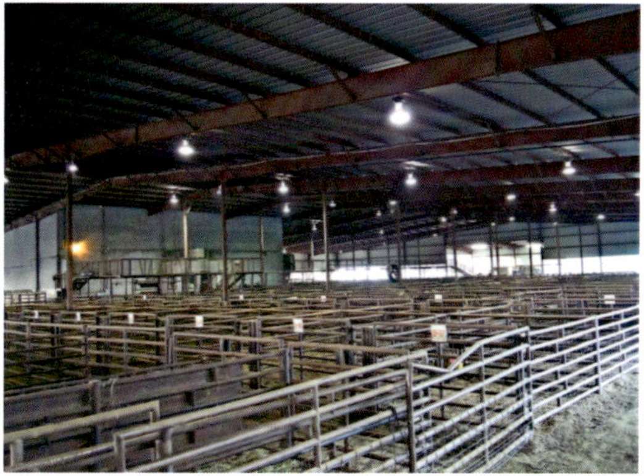

Figure 22. Auction markets expose naïve cattle to various pathogenic organisms, and cattle originating from auctions are more likely to develop BRDC. Image courtesy of Dr. Sarah Capik.

Clinical signs

- The correct diagnosis of BRDC is the most challenging aspect of the disease because the clinical signs are generally subjective and non-specific. One system uses a collection of clinical findings in acronym form as D.A.R.T. (depression, anorexia, respiration, temperature).[27] The observations that can be made in the pen or pasture are depression, loss of appetite (judged by rumen fill), abnormal respiration rate/character.
- A calf with these symptoms is further evaluated in a chute. While restrained, a complete examination can be performed, including auscultation of the lung fields, rumen motility and collection of rectal temperature.
- Many scoring systems have been developed using a scaling score of depression and respiration in conjunction with a threshold rectal temperature to diagnose BRDC in an individual calf.

- Signs of depression include reduced responsiveness, reluctance to move or stand unless approached closely, or moribund and unable to rise.
- Anorexia, or lack of rumen fill, is noticeable through a depression in the paralumbar fossa (also referred to as being gaunt).
- Respiratory scores are generally guided by the absence or presence of nasal and ocular discharge (its quantity and thickness), the rate of respiration, and the effort with which it is conducted (dyspnoea, orthopneic stance, open-mouth breathing or panting).
- A rectal temperature threshold of 40 °C is commonly used as a guide for treatment. Cattle displaying the other symptoms of disease with a rectal temperature ≥40 °C are diagnosed with BRDC and subsequently treated.

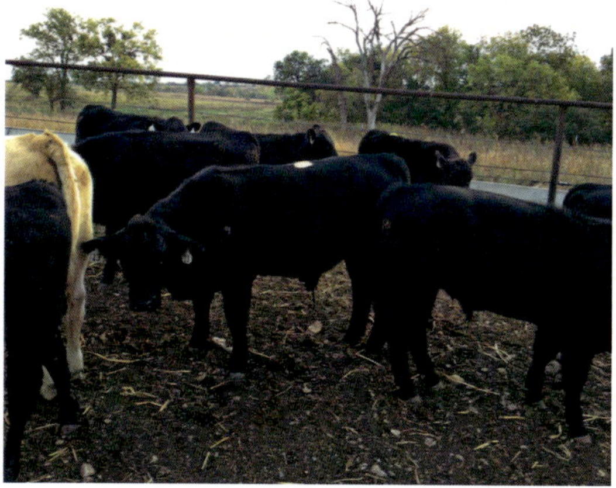

Figure 23. Depression: lowered ears, lowered head, glazed over eyes, weak and slow walking when stimulated to move.

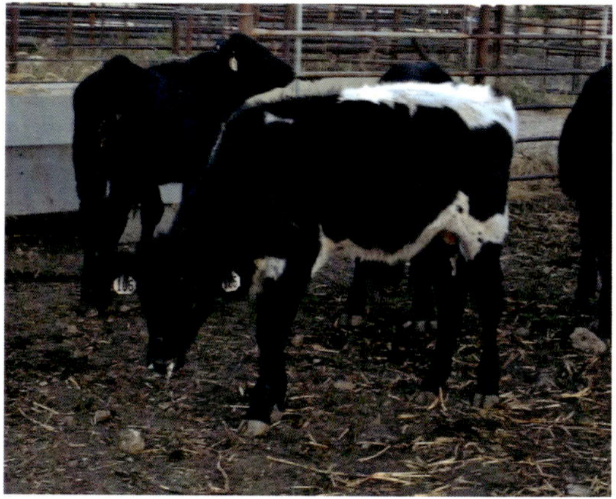

Figure 24. Severe depression with feet dragging or buckling at the joints due to weakness.

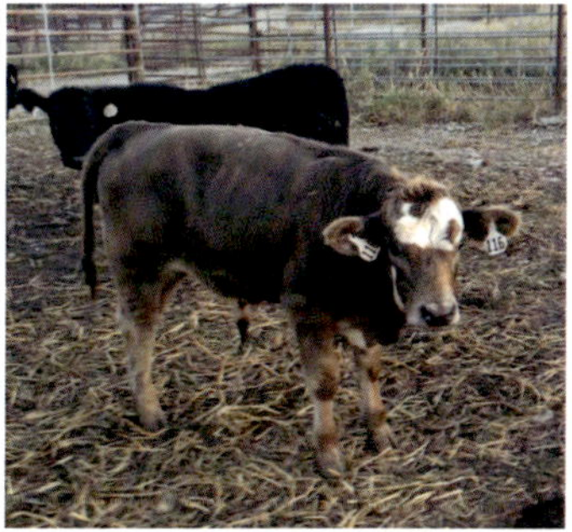

Figure 25. Anorexia: decrease or absence of an appetite can result in a sunken area at the paralumbar fossa due to lack of rumen fill.

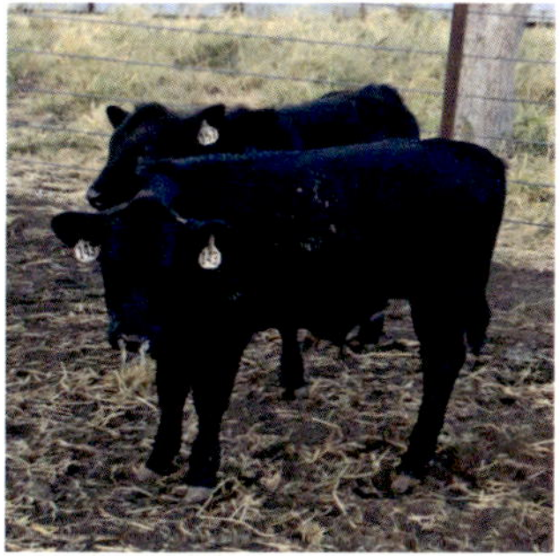

Figure 26. Respiration: thick purulent nasal discharge.

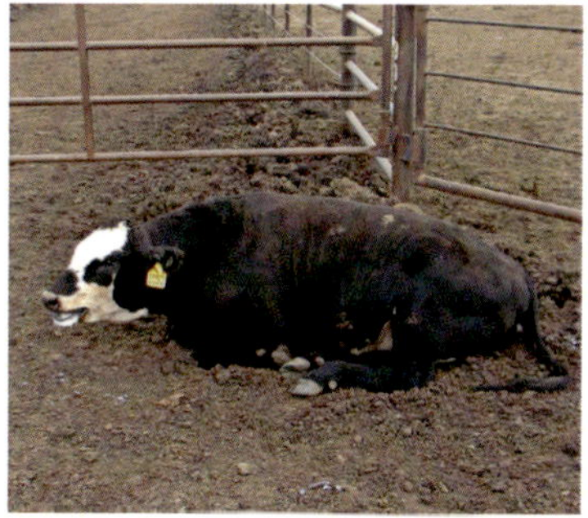

Figure 27. Respiration: the calf is recumbent and displaying dyspnoea and tachypnoea.

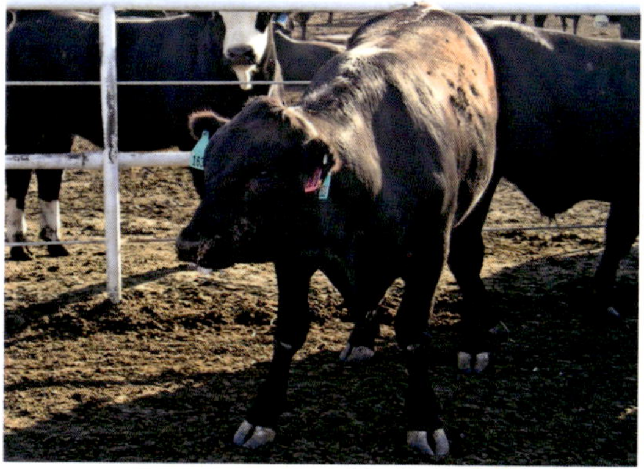

Figure 28. Respiration: orthopneic stance, head and neck extended, front legs spread to decrease thoracic pressure.

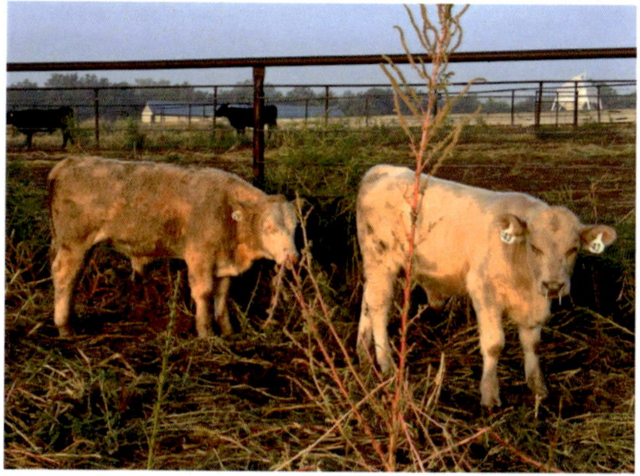

Figure 29. Two calves each displaying three of the cardinal signs of BRDC: depression, copious nasal discharge and anorexia.

- Researchers have made many attempts at more objective measures of BRDC diagnosis such as lung biopsy,[28] ultrasound,[3, 16, 29, 30] automated thermography,[31] biological markers,[32] and thoracic auscultation.[29, 33, 34] Some of these modalities have shown promise as diagnostic adjuncts but have not been widely accepted in the field.

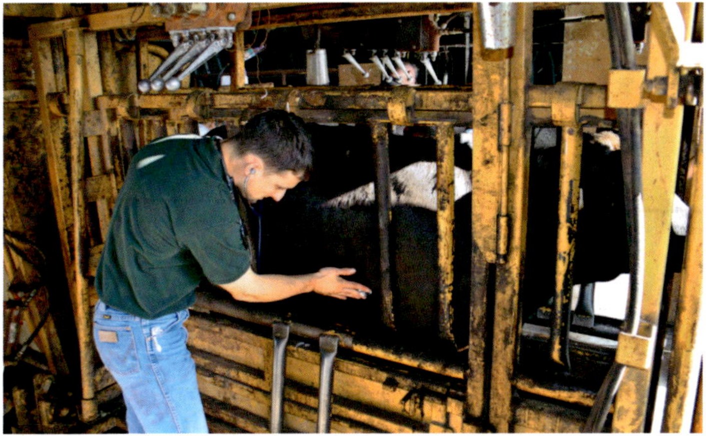

Figure 30. Veterinarian performing thoracic auscultation as a diagnostic tool.

Bacterial and viral diagnosis

When selecting animals for BRDC diagnostic testing, one should select them early in the disease process (within the first 2-3 days) and prior to any therapy. Diagnostic testing of animals displaying chronic disease or after therapy with antimicrobial treatments will yield results that are often inaccurate and hard to interpret due to secondary infections and the presence of antimicrobial resistance that may not be present in untreated cohorts. [35] Good clinical histories should be provided to the testing laboratory, and their assistance in guiding testing, handling, and shipping procedures should be sought.

Antemortem sampling

- Historically, nasal swabs (NS) were used in place of either transtracheal wash (TTW) or bronchoalveolar lavage fluid (BALF) in attempt to identify BRDC pathogens antemortem.[35] However, it has been demonstrated that nasopharyngeal swabs (NPS) can be moderately predictive of the bacteria present in the lung,[36, 37] and are a preferred diagnostic source.[16]
- To avoid contamination, use a double guarded swab for collection of NPS and thoroughly clean the nares prior to sampling. The swab is inserted in the nare, directed medial and ventrally until the point where resistance is met prior to retracting the guard from the swab.

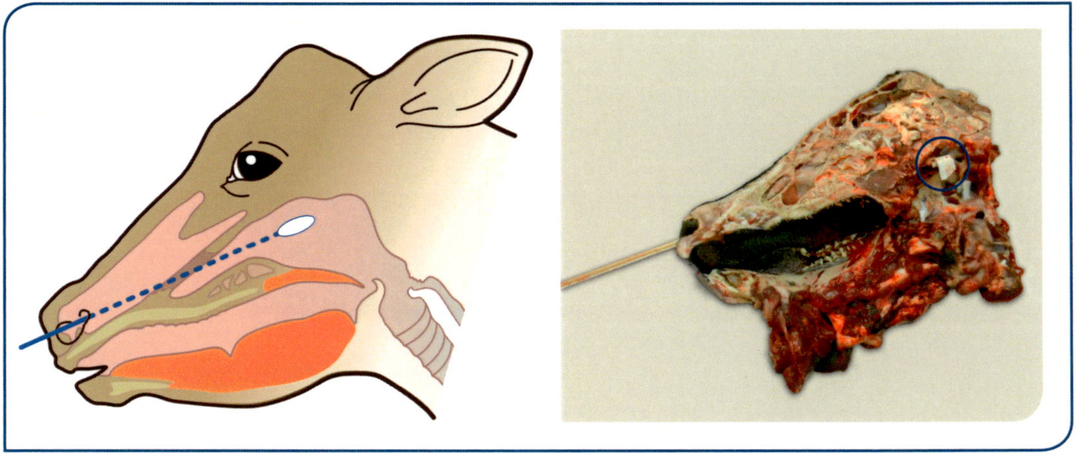

Figure 31. Placement of the swab, as illustrated, will result in a sample from the nasopharyngeal area.
Image courtesy of Dr. Sarah Capik.

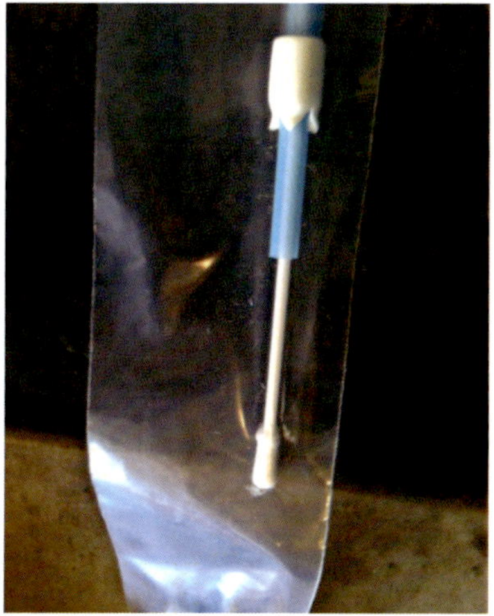

Figure 32. A double guarded swab (extended from its protectant sheath) is utilized to minimize contamination from the nares and nasal turbinates when collecting NPS samples.

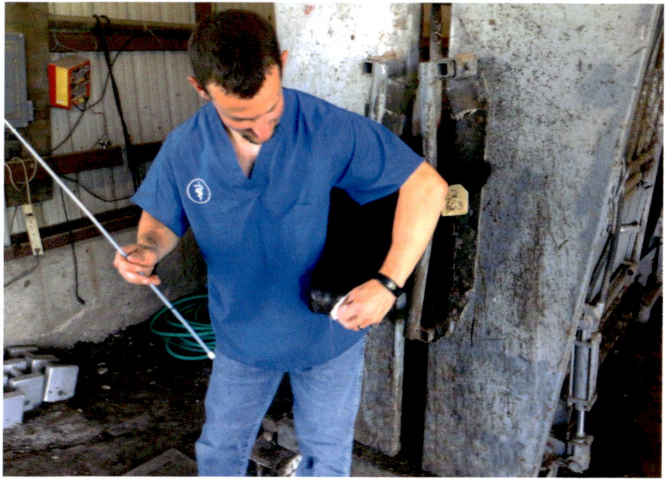

Figure 33. Purulent discharge and foreign material must be cleaned from the nare prior to inserting the swab.

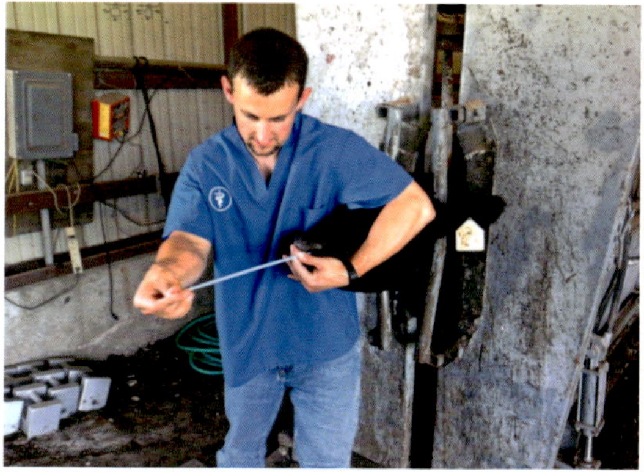

Figure 34. Restraint is accomplished either manually or with a rope halter to facilitate entry of the swab into the nasopharyngeal area.

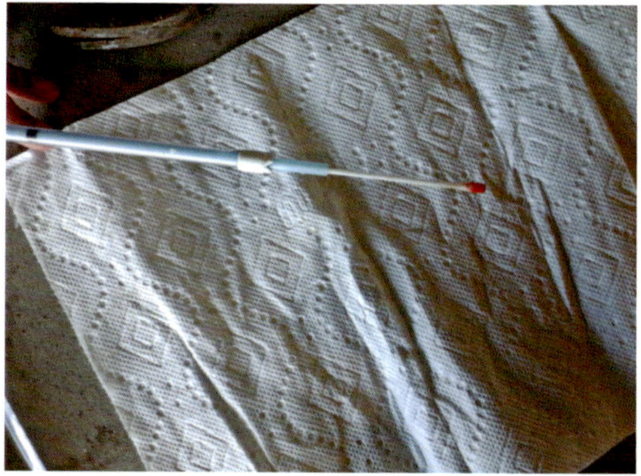

Figure 35. A small amount of blood on swab after NPS is normal.

- Another procedure involves the collection of BALF. While restraining the head in a vertical position, insert the tube ventral and medially into either nare, blindly, until resistance is met in the lung. The animal will often cough as it passes through the trachea. If using a bronchoalveolar tube, it is best to not inflate the cuff after placement, as this will create too much pressure and can cause either lung damage or backflow of fluid around the cuff, and minimal fluid will be obtained from the procedure.
- Although data on these procedures for viral testing are limited, it would seem a plausible mean for viral diagnosis as well.
- TTW is more invasive (skin incision and tracheal puncture) than BALF collection and not discussed further.

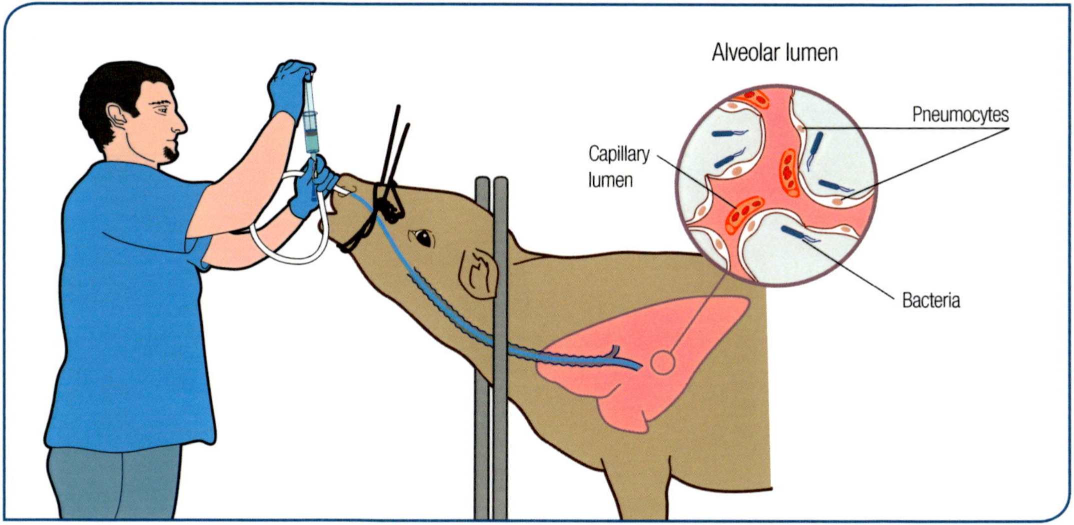

Figure 36. Sterile saline is directly deposited into the lung with immediate aspiration of fluid resulting in a good diagnostic sample. Centrifugation results in a cell pellet to be resuspended in liquid culture medium.

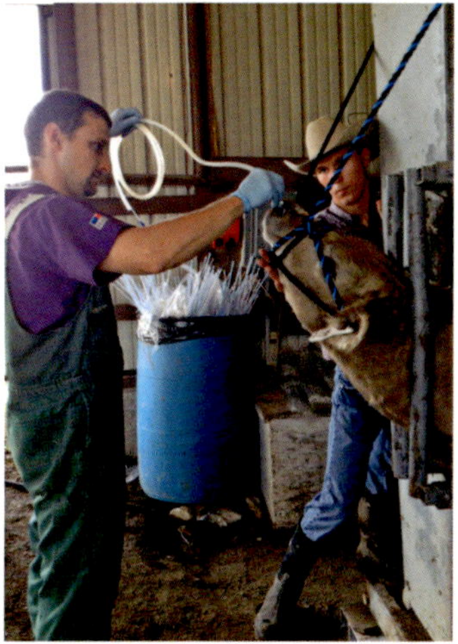

Figure 37. BALF collection procedure, restraining the head in a vertical position, allows passage of BAL tube access to trachea.

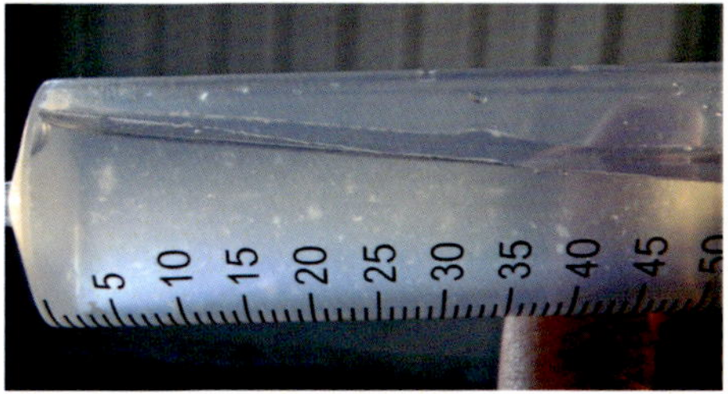

Figure 38. Fluid recovered following BALF collection, saline contains flecks of purulent material.

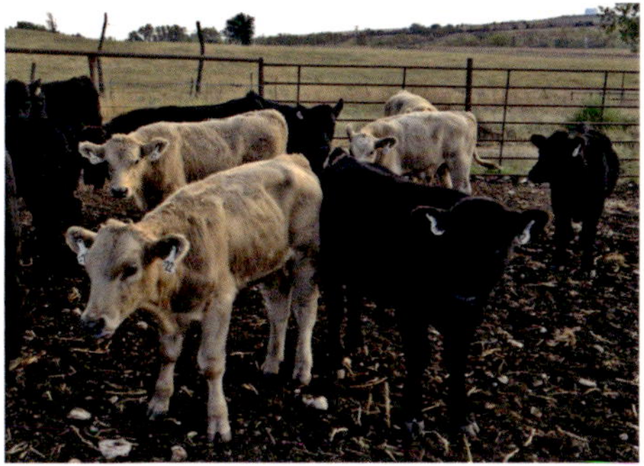

Figure 39. Antemortem inspection: animal displaying signs of chronic BRDC infection (weakness, dyspnoea and cachexy). Not a good source of diagnostic samples.

Postmortem sampling

Postmortem samples should ideally come from animals that have died from acute BRDC prior to treatment. Guidance should be sought from the diagnostic laboratory for suggested samples in a BRDC workup. However, general guidelines would include fresh and fixed (10 % formalin) lung from the junction of diseased and non-diseased lung, serum, tracheal and mesenteric lymph nodes, and an ear notch (testing for BVDV persistent infection).[9]

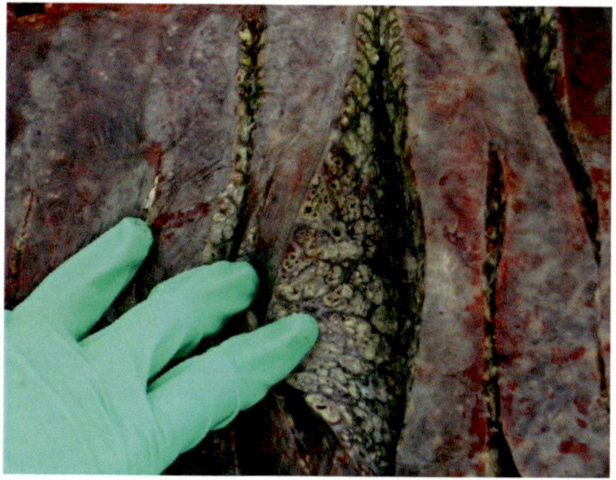

Figure 40. Chronic lesions of BRDC: lung is nearly 100 % consolidated and bronchioles are full of abscesses. Culturing these lesions will provide no diagnostic value.

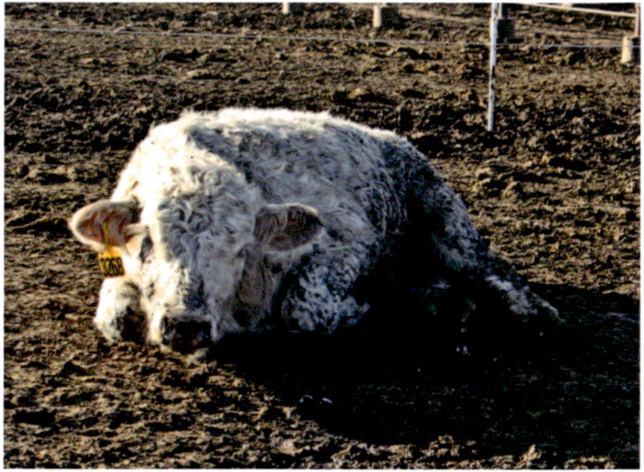

Figure 41. Cattle acutely moribund and unlikely to respond to therapy are a good source of diagnostic samples. Image courtesy of Dr. DJ Rezac and Beef Cattle Institute.

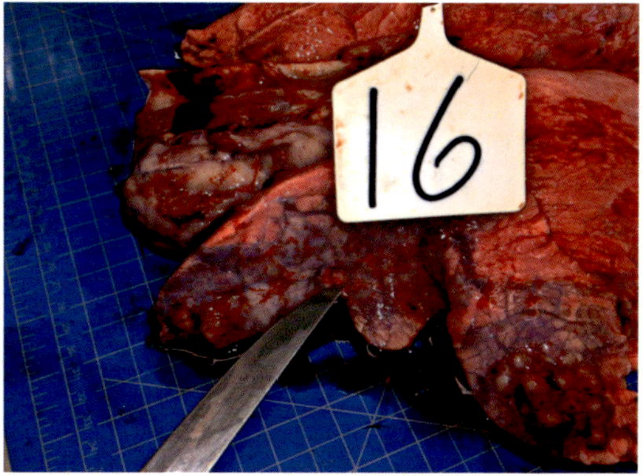

Figure 42. Acute BRDC lesions from animals not yet treated provide optimal diagnostic samples.

Antimicrobial therapy

- Following diagnosis of BRDC in an individual calf, antimicrobial therapy is the mainstay of treatment. Regulations regarding their use will vary by the country, and local regulations should always be consulted and followed by the veterinarian. In some countries, cattle at high risk for developing BRDC (young, highly stressed and often commingled) will allow prophylactic (i.e. metaphylaxis) administration of antimicrobials in attempt to control or suppress BRDC outbreaks.

- Specific pharmacology textbooks or formularies should be consulted for guidance in antimicrobial selection in specific cases. Generally, antimicrobial classes with a broad spectrum (e.g. macrolides, fluoroquinolones, phenicols, and cephalosporins) are preferred. One factor in antimicrobial selection will be considering the mechanism of action of the antimicrobial and the pathogen being treated. As discussed earlier, MB does not have a cell wall so antimicrobials targeting cell walls (e.g. penicillins, cephalosporins) will be ineffective.

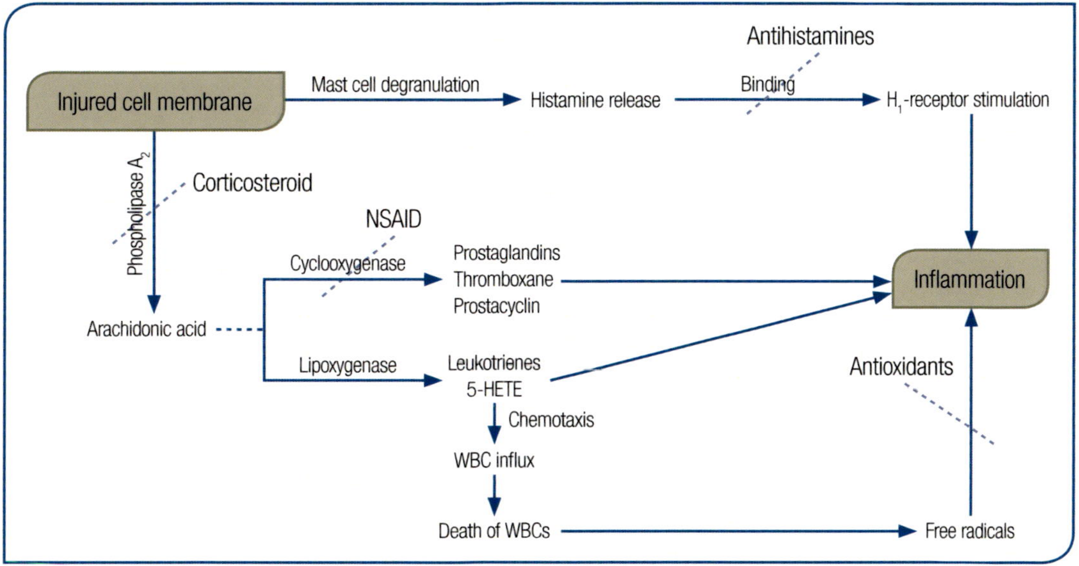

Figure 43. Site of action of some anti-inflammatory agents in the cellular inflammation cascade.

Antimicrobial resistance (AR)

- Another factor guiding antimicrobial selection is BRDC pathogen resistance. Monitoring trends in AR is currently a high priority to ensure that antimicrobial efficacy is maintained and to ensure that the risk of transferring AR from food producing animals to humans remains low.

- The VetPath study is an ongoing pan-European AR monitoring programme that collects pathogens from acute clinical BRDC cases prior to treatment. The most recent report shows very low levels of AR in the major antimicrobial classes. [16] Similar studies also report the same AR trends, finding AR to be low in the most commonly used antimicrobials (danofloxacin, enrofloxacin, tilmicosin, florfenicol, ceftiofur). [28, 37] However, AR to the tetracyclines, sulfonamides and spectinomycin are often reported to be higher. A word of caution must be again stated at the interpretation of AR reports from cattle that have chronic disease or have received prior treatment with an antimicrobial as AR tends to be higher in these animals. [35]

Ancillary therapy (AT)

- AT to antimicrobial treatment of BRDC is controversial. AT that is often used includes: NSAIDs, corticosteroids, antihistamines, injectable vitamins A, D, E and C. The goal of AT is to decrease severity of clinical signs, increase feed intake, and decrease the damage to the lung through decreased inflammation.[38]
- Currently, there are no studies that consistently support the use of NSAIDs as a viable AT in the treatment of BRDC.[38] In fact, NSAIDs have been recently shown to have detrimental effects in the treatment of BRDC.[39] Studies evaluating the use of dexamethasone (corticosteroid) have shown poorer therapeutic response, more relapses, and a longer duration of BRDC.[40] In regard to vitamin use in BRDC AT, one study reported that vitamin C reduced mortality rate. However, a recent study found it to provide no benefits.[39]
- In summation, the small amount of data on AT use in BRDC is conflicting and therefore, at this time AT is generally not recommended in treatment of BRDC.

Vaccination

Bacterial vaccination

- Vaccinating cattle against bacterial pathogens of BRDC has long been a debated clinical practice. The body of evidence supporting the use of bacterial vaccinations is small. In a meta-analysis on the benefits of using commercially available bacterial vaccines to decrease BRDC, researchers found a potential benefit for use of MH and PM vaccines but no benefit of HS vaccines.[41]
- There are several commercial bacterial vaccines available and their use should be determined on a case by case basis in veterinarian-client consultation.

Viral vaccination

Few studies have investigated the use of viral vaccines in a natural exposure trial. However, results from challenge studies and anecdotal field evidence suggest that it is an important part in the management of BRDC. Commercially available multivalent vaccines are recommended to be used according to the directions on the label.

Management

- Controlling factors related to management can be challenging due to availability of resources and practicality of implementation. However, some management practices are inexpensive and proven to work. Two such examples: ensuring the passage of maternal antibodies to the newborn calf and purchasing lower risk calves in feeding/fattening operations.

- Ensuring that a newborn calf nurse within 24 hours of birth transfers maternal antibodies to the newborn. The failure of passive transfer has been shown to triple the risk of BRDC. [42]

- In feeding/fattening operations, BRDC risk can be lessened by changing purchasing practices; single-source calves with a known history of vaccinations can lessen the risk of BRDC. [43]

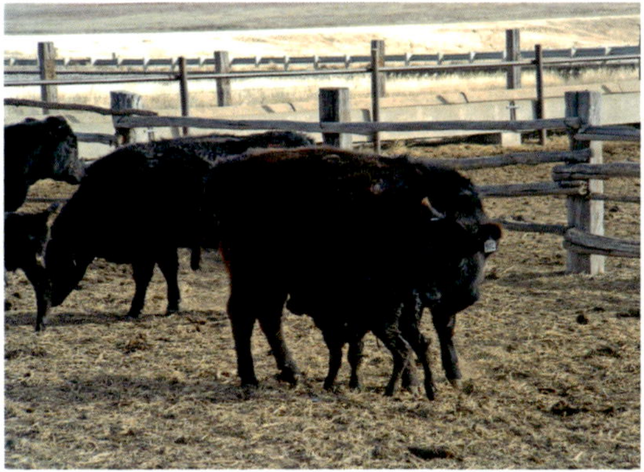

Figure 44. Ensuring that colostrum is ingested within the first 24 hours of life reduces the chance that a calf can get BRDC in the future. Image courtesy of Dr. DJ Rezac and Beef Cattle Institute.

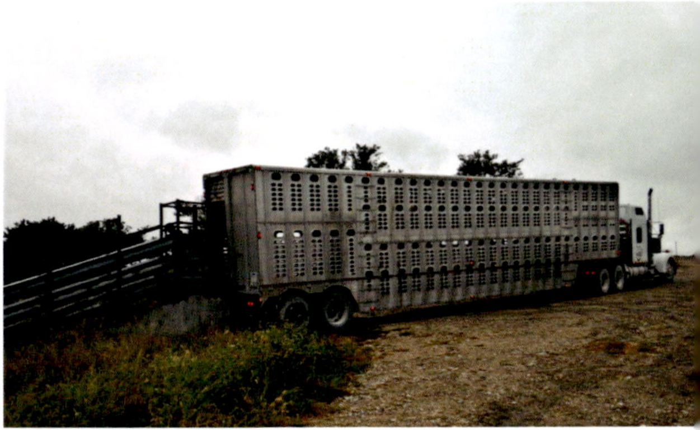

Figure 45. Avoiding auction markets and long transportation decreases the risk of BRDC.

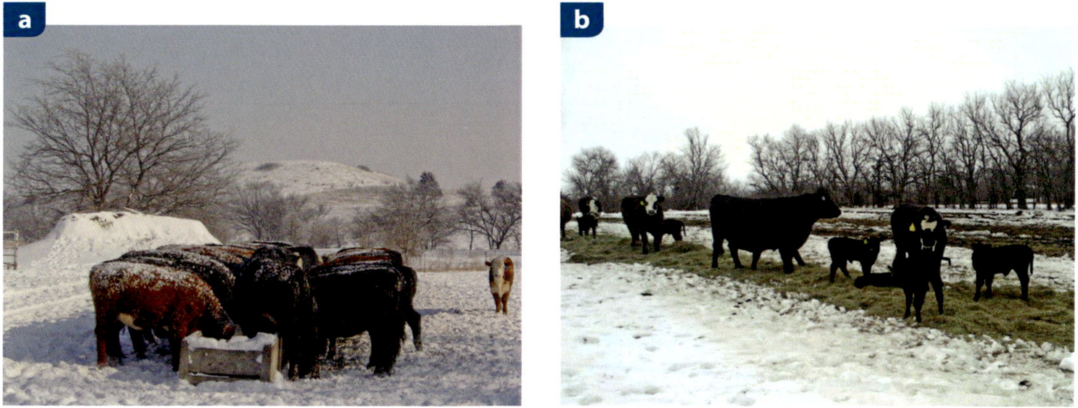

Figure 46. Ensuring good bedding and access to feed and water in times of weather extremes minimize stress. Images courtesy of Dr. DJ Rezac and Beef Cattle Institute (a), and Kelly DeDonder (b).

Conclusions

BRDC is a multifaceted and complex disease process. Strategies aimed to lessen the impact of BRDC begin at birth and continue throughout the life of the animal. The role of a veterinarian can serve many functions in this cycle. Maintaining a strong relationship with the producer will facilitate the early identification of management strategies that can be implemented to help reduce the effect of BRDC.

References

1. Watts, J.L., Sweeney, M.T. 2010. Antimicrobial resistance in bovine respiratory disease pathogens: measures, trends, and impact on efficacy. *Veterinary Clinics of North America: Food Animal Practice,* 26: 79-88, table of contents.
2. Hilton, W.M. 2014. BRD in 2014: where have we been, where are we now, and where do we want to go? *Animal Health Research Reviews,* 15: 120-122.
3. Flock, M. 2004. Diagnostic ultrasonography in cattle with thoracic disease. *The Veterinary Journal,* 167: 272-280.
4. Griebel, P., Hill, K., Stookey, J. 2014. How stress alters immune responses during respiratory infection. *Animal Health Research Reviews,* 15: 161-165.
5. Mosier, D. 2014. Review of BRD pathogenesis: the old and the new. *Animal Health Research Reviews,* 15: 166-168.
6. O'Neill, R., Mooney, J., Connaghan, E., Furphy, C., Graham, D.A. 2014. Patterns of detection of respiratory viruses in nasal swabs from calves in Ireland: a retrospective study. *Veterinary Record,* 175: 351.
7. Griffin, D., Chengappa, M.M., Kuszak, J., McVey, D.S. 2010. Bacterial pathogens of the bovine respiratory disease complex. *Veterinary Clinics of North America: Food Animal Practice,* 26: 381-394.
8. Ridpath, J. 2010. The contribution of infections with bovine viral diarrhea viruses to bovine respiratory disease. *Veterinary Clinics of North America: Food Animal Practice*, 26: 335-348.
9. Campbell, J.R. 2004. Effect of bovine viral diarrhea virus in the feedlot. *Veterinary Clinics of North America: Food Animal Practice,* 20: 39-50.
10. Paulsen, D. 2013. Respiratory diseases of cattle. American College of Veterinary Pathologists Annual Meeting.
11. Storz, J., Lin, X., Purdy, C.W., Chouljenko, V.N., Kousoulas, K.G., Enright, F.M., Gilmore, W.C., Briggs, R.E., Loan, R.W. 2000. Coronavirus and *Pasteurella* infections in bovine shipping fever pneumonia and Evans' criteria for causation. *Journal of Clinical Microbiology,* 38: 3291-3298.
12. Sandal, I., Inzana, T.J., Molinaro, A., De Castro, C., Shao, J.Q., Apicella, M.A., Cox, A.D., St Michael, F., Berg, G. 2011. Identification, structure, and characterization of an exopolysaccharide produced by *Histophilus somni* during biofilm formation. *BMC Microbiology,* 11: 186.
13. McDougald, D., Rice, S.A., Barraud, N., Steinberg, P.D., Kjelleberg, S. 2012. Should we stay or should we go: mechanisms and ecological consequences for biofilm dispersal. *Nature Reviews Microbiology,* 10: 39-50.
14. Clawson, M.L., Murray, R.W. 2014. Pathogen variation across time and space: sequencing to characterize *Mannheimia haemolytica* diversity. *Animal Health Research Reviews,* 15: 169-171.

15. Confer, A.W. 2009. Update on bacterial pathogenesis in BRD. *Animal Health Research Reviews,* 10: 145-148.
16. de Jong, A., Thomas, V., Simjee, S., Moyaert, H., El Garch, F., Maher, K., Morrissey, I., Butty, P., Klein, U., Marion, H., Rigaut, D., Vallé, M. 2014. Antimicrobial susceptibility monitoring of respiratory tract pathogens isolated from diseased cattle and pigs across Europe: the VetPath study. *Veterinary Microbiology,* 172: 202-215.
17. Gautier-Bouchardon, A.V., Ferre, S., Le Grand, D., Paoli, A., Gay, E., Poumarat, F. 2014. Overall decrease in the susceptibility of *Mycoplasma bovis* to antimicrobials over the past 30 years in France. *PLoS One,* 9: e87672.
18. Bürki, S., Frey, J., Pilo, P. 2015. Virulence, persistence and dissemination of *Mycoplasma bovis. Veterinary Microbiology,* 179: 15-22.
19. Kapil, S., Basaraba, R.J. 1997. Infectious bovine rhinotracheitis, parainfluenza-3, and respiratory coronavirus. *Veterinary Clinics of North America: Food Animal Practice,* 13: 455-469.
20. Klima, C.L., Alexander, T.W., Hendrick, S., McAllister, T.A. 2014. Characterization of *Mannheimia haemolytica* isolated from feedlot cattle that were healthy or treated for bovine respiratory disease. *Canadian Journal of Veterinary Research,* 78: 38-45.
21. Briggs, R.E., Frank, G.H., Purdy, C.W., Zehr, E.S., Loan, R.W. 1998. Rapid spread of a unique strain of *Pasteurella haemolytica* serotype 1 among transported calves. *American Journal of Veterinary Research,* 59: 401-405.
22. Timsit, E., Christensen, H., Bareille, N., Seegers, H., Bisgaard, M., Assié, S. 2013. Transmission dynamics of *Mannheimia haemolytica* in newly-received beef bulls at fattening operations. *Veterinary Microbiology,* 161: 295-304.
23. Taylor, J.D., Fulton, R.W., Dabo, S.M., Lehenbauer, T.W., Confer, A.W. 2010. Comparison of genotypic and phenotypic characterization methods for *Pasteurella multocida* isolates from fatal cases of bovine respiratory disease. *Journal of Veterinary Diagnostic Investigation,* 22: 366-375.
24. Taylor, J.D., Fulton, R.W., Lehenbauer, T.W., Step, D.L., Confer, A.W. 2010. The epidemiology of bovine respiratory disease: What is the evidence for predisposing factors? *Canadian Journal of Veterinary Research,* 51: 1095-1102.
25. Gay, E., Barnouin, J. 2009. A nation-wide epidemiological study of acute bovine respiratory disease in France. *Preventive Veterinary Medicine,* 89: 265-271.

26. Woolums, A.R., Berghaus, R.D., Smith, D.R., White, B.J., Engelken, T.J., Irsik, M.B., Matlick, D.K., Jones, A.L., Ellis, R.W., Smith, I.J., Mason, G.L., Waggoner, E.R. 2013. Producer survey of herd-level risk factors for nursing beef calf respiratory disease. *Journal of the American Veterinary Medical Association,* 243: 538-547.
27. Griffin, D. 2014. The monster we don't see: subclinical BRD in beef cattle. *Animal Health Research Reviews,* 15: 138-141.
28. Wallmann, J., Kaspar, H., Kroker, R. 2004. Data on the prevalence of antimicrobial susceptibility of veterinary pathogens from cattle and pigs: national antibiotic resistance monitoring 2002/2003 of the BVL. *Berliner Und Munchener Tierarztliche Wochenschrift,* 117: 480-492.
29. Kadlec, K., von Czapiewski, E., Kaspar, H., Wallmann, J., Michael, G.B., Steinacker, U., Schwarz, S. 2011. Molecular basis of sulfonamide and trimethoprim resistance in fish-pathogenic *Aeromonas* isolates. *Applied and Environmental Microbiology,* 77: 7147-7150.
30. Buczinski, S., L Ollivett, T., Dendukuri, N. 2015. Bayesian estimation of the accuracy of the calf respiratory scoring chart and ultrasonography for the diagnosis of bovine respiratory disease in pre-weaned dairy calves. *Preventive Veterinary Medicine,* 119: 227-231.
31. Kaspar, H., Heidemanns, K., Roemer, A., Wallmann, J., Steinacker, U., Mankertz, J. 2012. Aquaculture as an impact factor for antimicrobial resistance: What do we know so far? Results of the German National Antibiotic Resistance Monitoring (GERM-Vet). *International Journal of Medical Microbiology,* 302: 144-144.
32. Plešková, V., Kašparovský, T., Obořil, M., Ptáčková, N., Chaloupková, R., Ladislav, D., Damborský, J., Lochman, J. 2011. Elicitin-membrane interaction is driven by a positive charge on the protein surface: role of Lys13 residue in lipids loading and resistance induction. *Plant Physiology and Biochemistry,* 49: 321-328.
33. DeDonder, K.D., Thomson, D.U., Loneragan, G.H. et al. 2010. Lung auscultation and rectal temperature as a predictor of lung lesions and bovine respiratory disease treatment outcome in feedyard cattle. *Bovine Practitioner,* 44: 146-153.
34. Noffsinger, T., Brattain, K., Quakenbush, G., Taylor, G. 2014. Field results from Whisper® stethoscope studies. *Animal Health Research Reviews,* 15: 142-144.
35. Hendriksen, R.S., Mevius, D.J., Schroeter, A., Teale, C., Meunier, D., Butaye, P., Franco, A., Utinane, A., Amado, A., Moreno, M., Greko, C., Stärk, K., Berghold, C., Myllyniemi, A.L., Wasyl, D., Sunde, M., Aarestrup, F.M. 2008. Prevalence of antimicrobial resistance among bacterial pathogens isolated from cattle in different European countries: 2002-2004. *Acta Vet Scand,* 50.
36. Cusack, P.M., McMeniman, N.P., Lean, I.J. 2008. Effects of injectable vitamins A, D, E and C on the health and growth rate of feedlot cattle destined for the Australian domestic market. *Australian Veterinary Journal,* 86: 81-87.

37. Kaspar, H., Roemer, A., Steinacker, U., Wallmann, J. 2011. The German National Antibiotic Resistance Monitoring (GERM-Vet): results of veterinary pathogens from cattle over a period of five years. *Veterinary Microbiology.*
38. Francoz, D., Buczinski, S., Apley, M. 2012. Evidence related to the use of ancillary drugs in bovine respiratory disease (anti-inflammatory and others): are they justified or not? *Veterinary Clinics of North America: Food Animal Practice,* 28: 23-38, vii-viii.
39. Wilson, B.K., Step, D.L., Maxwell, C.L., Wagner, J.J., Richards, C.J., Krehbiel, C.R. 2015. Evaluation of multiple ancillary therapies used in combination with an antimicrobial in newly received high-risk calves treated for bovine respiratory disease. *Journal of Animal Science.*
40. Christie, B.M., Pierson, R.E., Braddy, P.M., Flack, D.E., Horton, D.P., Jensen, R., Lee, E.A., Remmenga, E.E., Rutt, K.G. 1977. Efficacy of corticosteroids as supportive therapy for bronchial pneumonia in yearling feedlot cattle. *Bovine Practitioner,* 12: 115-117.
41. Larson, R.L., Step, D.L. 2012. Evidence-based effectiveness of vaccination against *Mannheimia haemolytica, Pasteurella multocida,* and *Histophilus somni* in feedlot cattle for mitigating the incidence and effect of bovine respiratory disease complex. *Veterinary Clinics of North America: Food Animal Practice,* 28: 97-106, 106e101-107, ix.
42. Wittum, T.E., Perino, L.J. 1995. Passive immune status at postpartum hour 24 and long-term health and performance of calves. *American Journal of Veterinary Research,* 56: 1149-1154.
43. Edwards, T.A. 2010. Control methods for bovine respiratory disease for feedlot cattle. *Veterinary Clinics of North America: Food Animal Practice,* 26: 273-284.